BREAKFAST RECIPES 2021

Healthy and easy to prepare recipes for a special breakfast

Sommario

INTRODUCTION

The Mediterranean Diet constitutes a set of knowledge and traditions ranging from landscape to table, including crops, harvesting, fishing, conservation, processing, preparation, and consumption of food.

It is characterized by a nutritional model that has remained constant in time and places, being mainly made up of: olive oil, cereals, fresh and dried fruits, vegetables, a moderate amount of fish, dairy products, meat, many seasonings, and spices, entirely accompanied by wine. It is a model of a sustainable diet, as it contributes to preserve: quality, food, and nutritional safety and at the same time promotes the management of environmental and territorial resources.

Mediterranean diet is a specific diet by removing processed foods and high in saturated fats. It's not necessarily about losing weight, but rather a healthy lifestyle choice. It is about ingesting traditional ingredients consumed by those who have lived in the Mediterranean basin for a long time. This is a diet rich in fruits, vegetables, and fish. Cooking with olive oil is a fundamental ingredient and is an ideal replacement for saturated fats. Studies show that the people who live in these regions live longer and better lives.

CHAPTER 1: BREAKFAST RECIPES

Cheesy Caprese Style Portobellos Mushrooms

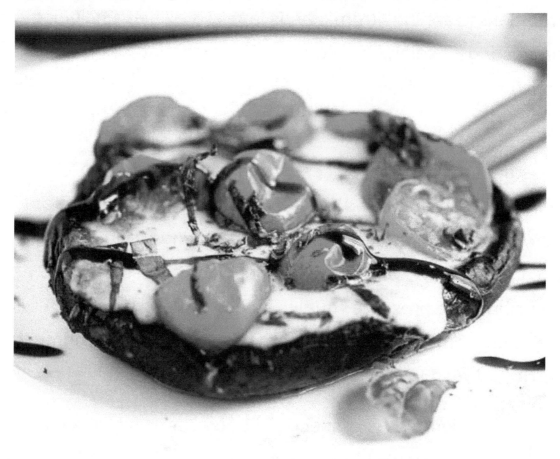

Servings: 2

Preparation time: 20 minutes

INGREDIENTS

2 large caps of Portobello mushroom, gills removed

4 tomatoes, halved

Salt and freshly cracked black pepper to taste

¼ cup fresh basil

4 tbsp olive oil

¼ cup shredded Mozzarella cheese

INSTRUCTIONS

1. Switch on the oven, then set its temperature to 400°F and let it preheat.

2. Place tomatoes in a bowl, season with salt and black pepper, add basil, drizzle with oil and toss until mixed.

3. Distribute cheese evenly in the bottom of each mushroom cap and then top with prepared tomato mixture.

4. Take a baking sheet, line it with aluminum foil, place prepared mushrooms on it and bake for some minutes until thoroughly cooked.

5. Serve straight away.

   NUTRITION Calories 315, Total Fat 29.2g, Total Carbs 14.2g, Protein 4.7g, Sugar 10.4g, Sodium 55mg

Pear Oatmeal

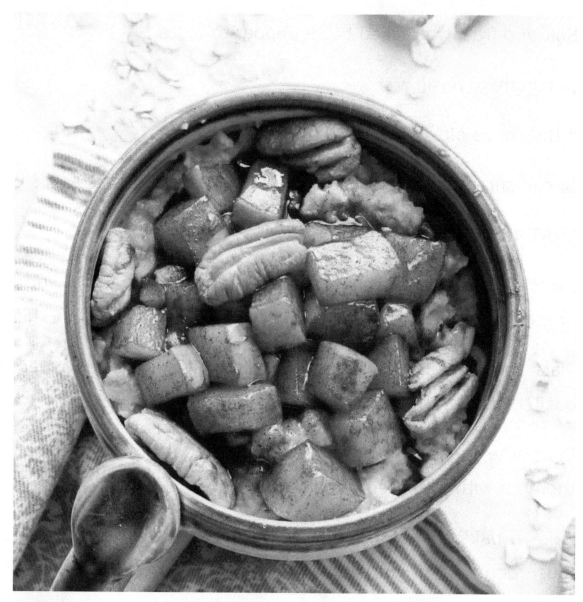

Servings: 4

Preparation time: 25 minutes

INGREDIENTS

1 cup oatmeal

1/3 cup milk

1 pear, chopped

1 teaspoon vanilla extract

1 tablespoon Splenda

1 teaspoon butter

½ teaspoon ground cinnamon

1 egg, beaten

DIRECTIONS

1. In the big bowl, mix up together oatmeal, milk, egg, vanilla extract, Splenda, and ground cinnamon.

2. Melt butter and add it to the oatmeal mixture.

3. Then add chopped pear and stir it well.

4. Transfer the oatmeal mixture to the casserole mold and flatten gently. Cover it with foil and secure edges.

5. Bake the oatmeal for 25 minutes at 350F.

   NUTRITION Calories 151, Fat 3.9g, Fiber 3.3g, Carbs 23.6g, Protein 4.9g

Mediterranean Frittata

Servings: 6

Preparation time: 15 minutes

INGREDIENTS

- 9 large eggs, lightly beaten

- 8 kalamata olives, pitted, chopped

- ¼ cup olive oil

- 1/3 cup parmesan cheese, freshly grated

- 1/3 cup fresh basil, thinly sliced

- ½ teaspoon salt

- ½ teaspoon pepper

- ½ cup onion, chopped

- 1 sweet red pepper, diced

- 1 medium zucchini, cut to 1/2-inch cubes

- 1 package (4 ounces) feta cheese, crumbled

DIRECTIONS

1. In a 10-inch oven-proof skillet, heat the olive oil until hot. Add the olives, zucchini, red pepper, and onions, constantly stirring, until the vegetables are tender.

2. In a bowl, mix the eggs, feta cheese, basil, salt, and pepper; pour in the skillet with vegetables. Adjust heat to medium-low, cover, and cook for some minutes, or until the egg mixture is almost set.

3. Remove from the heat and sprinkle with the parmesan cheese. Transfer to the broiler.

4. With the oven door partially open, broil 5 ½ from the source of heat for about 2-3 minutes or until the top is golden. Cut into wedges.

NUTRITIONAL Calories 288.5, Fat 22.8g, Chol 301mg, Sodium 656 mg, Carb 5.6g, Fiber 1.2g, Sugar 3.3g, Protein 15.2g

Mediterranean Egg Casserole

Servings: 8

Preparation time: 50 minutes

INGREDIENTS

- 1 ½ cups (6 ounces) feta cheese, crumbled

- 1 jar (6 ounces) marinated artichoke hearts, drained well, coarsely chopped

- 10 eggs

- 2 cups milk, low-fat

- 2 cups fresh baby spinach, packed, coarsely chopped

- 6 cups whole-wheat baguette, cut into i-inch cubes

- 1 tablespoon garlic (about 4 cloves), finely chopped

- 1 tablespoon olive oil, extra-virgin

- ½ cup red bell pepper, chopped

- ½ cup Parmesan cheese, shredded

- ½ teaspoon pepper

- ½ teaspoon red pepper flakes

- ½ teaspoon salt

- 1/3 cup kalamata olives, pitted, halved

- ¼ cup red onion, chopped

- ¼ cup tomatoes (sun-dried) in oil, drained, chopped

DIRECTIONS

1. Preheat oven to 350 F.

2. Grease a 9x13 inch baking dish with olive oil cooking spray.

3. In an 8-inch non-stick pan over medium heat, heat the olive oil. Add the onions, garlic, and bell pepper; cook for about 3 minutes, frequently stirring, until slightly softened. Add the spinach; cook for about 1 minute or until starting to wilt.

4. Layer half of the baguette cubes in the prepared baking dish, then 1 cup of the feta, 1/4 cup Parmesan, the bell pepper mix, artichokes, the olives, and the tomatoes. Top with the remaining baguette cubes and then with the remaining ½ cup of feta.

5. In a large mixing bowl, whisk the eggs and the low-fat milk together. Beat in the pepper, salt, and pepper. Pour the mix over the bread layer in the baking dish, slightly pressing down. Sprinkle with the remaining ¼ cup Parmesan.

6. Bake for about 40-45 minutes, or until the center is set and the top is golden brown. Before serving, let stand for 15 minutes.

NUTRITION Calories 360, Fat 21g, Chol 270mg, Sodium 880mg, Carb 24g, Fiber 3g, Sugar 7g, Protein 20g

Egg Casserole with Paprika

Servings: 4

Preparation time: 40 minutes

INGREDIENTS

- 2 eggs, beaten

- 1 red bell pepper, chopped

- 1 chili pepper, chopped

- ½ red onion, diced

- 1 teaspoon canola oil

- ½ teaspoon salt

- 1 teaspoon paprika

- 1 tablespoon fresh cilantro, chopped

- 1 garlic clove, diced

- 1 teaspoon butter, softened

- ¼ teaspoon chili flakes

DIRECTIONS

Brush the casserole mold with canola oil and pour beaten eggs inside.

After this, toss the butter in the skillet and melt it over medium heat.

Add chili pepper and red bell pepper.

After this, add red onion and cook the vegetables for 7-8 minutes over medium heat. Stir them from time to time.

Transfer the vegetables to the casserole mold.

Add salt, paprika, cilantro, diced garlic, and chili flakes. Stir gently with the help of a spatula to get a homogenous mixture.

Bake the casserole for no minutes at 355F in the oven.

Then chill the meal well and cut into servings. Transfer the casserole to the serving plates with the help of the spatula.

NUTRITION: Calories 168, Fat 12,3, Fiber 1.5g, Carbs 4 4g, Protein 8.8g

Paprika Salmon Toast

Servings: 2

Preparation time: 3 minutes

INGREDIENTS

- 4 whole-grain bread slices

- 2 oz smoked salmon, sliced

- 2 teaspoons cream cheese

- 1 teaspoon fresh dill, chopped

- ½ teaspoon lemon juice

- ½ teaspoon paprika

- 4 lettuce leaves

- 1 cucumber, sliced

DIRECTIONS

Toast the bread in the toaster (1-2 minutes totally).

In the bowl, mix up together fresh dill, cream cheese, lemon juice, and paprika.

Then spread the toasts with the cream cheese mixture.

Slice the smoked salmon and place it on bread slices.

Add sliced cucumber and lettuce leaves.

Top the lettuce with remaining bread toasts and pin with the toothpick.

NUTRITION Calories 202, Fat 4.7g, Fiber 5.1g, Carbs 31.5g, Protein 12.7g

Scrambled Eggs

Servings: 2

Preparation time: 10 minutes

INGREDIENTS

- 1 yellow bell pepper, chopped

- 8 cherry tomatoes, cubed

- 2 spring onions, chopped

- 1 tablespoon olive oil

- 1 tablespoon capers, drained

- 2 tablespoons black olives, pitted and sliced

- 4 eggs

- A pinch of salt and black pepper

- ¼ teaspoon oregano, dried

- 1 tablespoon parsley, chopped

DIRECTIONS

1. Heat up a pan with the oil over medium-high heat, add the bell pepper and spring onions and sauté for 3 minutes.

2. Add the tomatoes, capers, and olives and sauté for a minute.

3. Crack the eggs into the pan, add salt, pepper, oregano, and scramble for 5 minutes more.

4. Divide the scramble between plates, sprinkle the parsley on top, and serve.

NUTRITION Calories 249, Fat 17g, Fiber 3.2g, Carbs 13.3g, Protein 13.5g

Cheesy Olives Bread

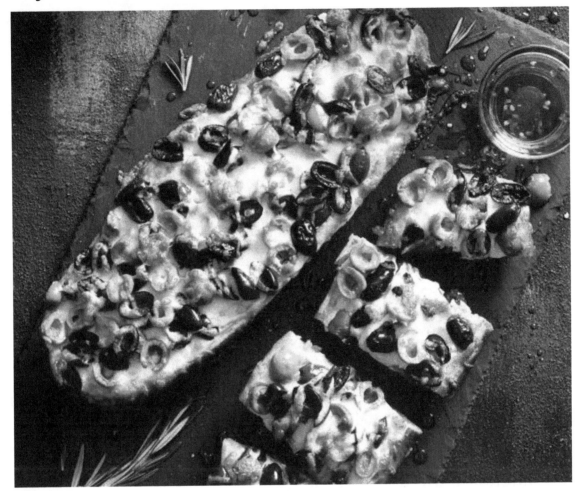

Servings: 10

Preparation time: 30 minutes

INGREDIENTS

4 cups whole-wheat flour

3 tablespoons oregano, chopped

2 teaspoons dry yeast

¼ cup olive oil

1 and ½ cups black olives, pitted and sliced

1 cup water

½ cup feta cheese, crumbled

DIRECTIONS

1. In a bowl, mix the flour with the water, the yeast, and the oil, stir, and knead your dough very well.

2. Put the dough in a bowl, cover with plastic wrap and keep in a warm place for 1 hour.

3. Divide the dough into 2 bowls and stretch each ball really well.

4. Add the rest of the ingredients on each ball and tuck them inside, well kneading the dough again.

5. Flatten the balls a bit and leave them aside for 4 minutes more.

6. Transfer the balls to a baking sheet lined with parchment paper, make a small slit in each, and bake at 425 degrees F for 30 minutes.

7. Serve the bread as a Mediterranean breakfast.

NUTRITION Calories 251, Fat 7.3g, Fiber 2.1g, Carbs 39.7g, Protein 6.7g

Mediterranean Freezer Breakfast Wraps

Servings: 4

Preparation time: 3 minutes

INGREDIENTS

1 cup spinach leaves, fresh, chopped

1 tablespoon water or low-fat milk

½ teaspoon garlic-chipotle seasoning or your preferred seasoning

4 eggs, beaten

4 pieces (8-inch) whole-wheat tortillas

4 tablespoons tomato chutney (or dried tomatoes, chopped or calmed tomatoes)

4 tablespoons feta cheese, crumbled (or goat cheese)

Optional: prosciutto, chopped or bacon, cooked, crumbled

Salt and pepper to taste

DIRECTIONS

1. In a mixing bowl, whisk the eggs, water, or milk, and seasoning together.

2. Heat a skillet with a little olive oil; pour the eggs and scramble for about 3-4 minutes, or until just cooked.

3. Lay the tortillas on a clean surface; divide the eggs between them, arranging the scrambled eggs, and leave the tortilla edges free to fold later.

4. Top the egg layer with about 1 tablespoon of cheese, 1 tablespoon of tomatoes, and 1/ 4 cup spinach. If using, layer with prosciutto or bacon.

5. In a burrito-style, roll up the tortillas, folding both of the ends in the process.

6. In a panini maker or a clean skillet, cook for about 1 minute, turning once, until the tortilla wraps are crisp and brown; serve.

NUTRITION Calories 450, Fat 15g, Chol 220mg, Sodium 280mg, Pot. 960mg, Carb 64g, Fiber 6g, Sugar 20g, Protein 17g

Milk Scones

Servings: 4

Preparation time: 10 minutes

INGREDIENTS

- ½ cup wheat flour, whole grain

- 1 teaspoon baking powder

- 1 tablespoon butter, melted

- 1 teaspoon vanilla extract

- 1 egg, beaten

- ¾ teaspoon salt

- 3 tablespoons milk

- 1 teaspoon vanilla sugar

DIRECTIONS

1. In the mixing bowl, combine together wheat flour, baking powder, butter, vanilla extract, and egg. Add salt and knead the soft and non-sticky dough. Add more flour if needed.

2. Then make the log from the dough and cut it into triangles.

3. Line the tray with baking paper.

4. Arrange the dough triangles on the baking paper and transfer them to the preheat to the 360F oven.

5. Cook the scones for 10 minutes or until they are light brown.

6. Then chill the scones and brush with milk and sprinkle with vanilla sugar.

NUTRITION Calories 112, Fat 4.4g, Fiber 0.5g, Carbs 14.3g, Protein 3.4g

Herbed Eggs and Mushroom Mix

Servings: 4

Preparation time: 20 minutes

INGREDIENTS

- 1 red onion, chopped

- 1 bell pepper, chopped

- 1 tablespoon tomato paste

- 1/3 cup water

- ½ teaspoon of sea salt

- 1 tablespoon butter

- 1 cup cremini mushrooms, chopped

- 1 tablespoon fresh parsley

- 1 tablespoon fresh dill

- 1 teaspoon dried thyme

- ½ teaspoon dried oregano

- ½ teaspoon paprika

- ½ teaspoon chili flakes

- ½ teaspoon garlic powder

- 4 eggs

DIRECTIONS

1. Toss butter in the pan and melt it.

2. Then add chopped mushrooms and bell pepper.

3. Roast the vegetables for 5 minutes over medium heat.

4. Then add onion and stir well.

5. Sprinkle the ingredients with garlic powder, chili flakes, dried oregano, and dried thyme. Mix up well

6. Then add tomato paste and water.

7. Mix up the mixture until it is homogenous.

8. Then add fresh parsley and dill.

9. Cook the mixture for 5 minutes over medium-high heat with the closed lid.

10.   After this, stir the mixture with the help of the spatula well.

11.   Crack the eggs over the mixture and close the lid.

12.   Cook for 10 minutes over low heat.

NUTRITION Calories 123, Fat 7.5g, Fiber 1.7g, Carbs 7.8, Protein 7.1g

Leeks and Eggs Muffins

Servings: 2

Preparation time: 20 minutes

INGREDIENTS

3 eggs, whisked

¼ cup baby spinach

2 tablespoons leeks, chopped

4 tablespoons parmesan, grated

2 tablespoons almond milk

Cooking spray

1 small red bell pepper, chopped

Salt and black pepper to the taste

1 tomato, cubed

2 tablespoons cheddar cheese, grated

DIRECTIONS

1. In a bowl, combine the eggs with the milk, salt, pepper, and the rest of the ingredients except the cooking spray and whisk well.

2. Grease a muffin tin with the cooking spray and divide the egg mixture in each muffin mould.

3. Bake at 380 degrees F for no minutes and serve them for breakfast.

   NUTRITION Calories 308, Fat 19.4g, Fiber 1.7g, Carbs 8.7g, Protein 24.4g

Mango and Spinach Bowls

Servings: 4

Preparation time: 0 minutes

INGREDIENTS

- 1 cup baby arugula

- 1 cup baby spinach, chopped

- 1 mango, peeled and cubed

- 1 cup strawberries, halved

- 1 tablespoon hemp seeds

- 1 cucumber, sliced

- 1 tablespoon lime juice

- 1 tablespoon tahini paste

- 1 tablespoon water

DIRECTIONS

In a salad bowl, mix the arugula with the rest of the ingredients except the tahini and the water and toss.

In a small bowl, combine the tahini with the water, whisk well, add to the salad, toss, divide into small bowls and serve for breakfast.

NUTRITION Calories 211, Fat 4.5g, Fiber 6.5g, Carbs 10.2g, Protein 3.5g

Figs Oatmeal

Servings: 5

Preparation time: 20 minutes

INGREDIENTS

- 2 cups oatmeal

- 1 ½ cup milk

- 1 tablespoon butter

- 3 figs, chopped

- 1 tablespoon honey

DIRECTIONS

1. Pour milk into the saucepan.

2. Add oatmeal and close the lid.

3. Cook the oatmeal for 15 minutes over medium-low heat.

4. Then add chopped figs and honey.

5. Add butter and mix up the oatmeal well.

6. Cook it for 5 minutes more.

7. Close the lid and let the cooked breakfast rest for 10 minutes before serving.

   NUTRITION Calories 222, Fat 6, Fiber 4.4g, carbs 36.5g, Protein 7.1g

Roasted Asparagus with Prosciutto and Poached Egg

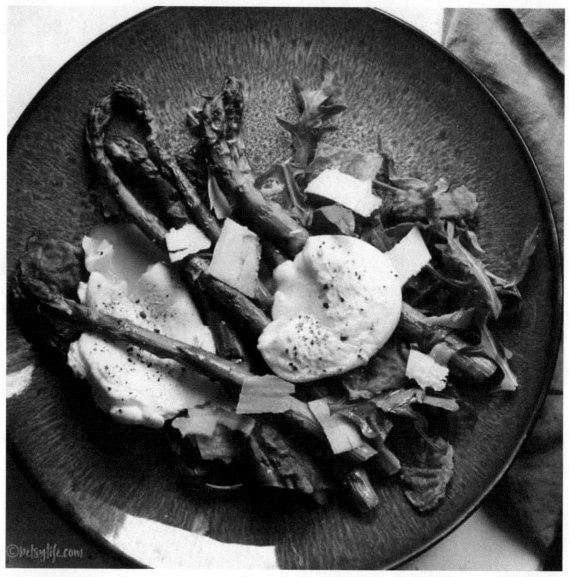

Servings: 4

Preparation time: 25 minutes

INGREDIENTS

- 1 bunch fresh asparagus, trimmed

- 1 tablespoon extra-virgin olive oil

- 4 eggs

- 2 ounces minced prosciutto

- ½ lemon, zested and juiced

- 1 tablespoon olive oil

- 1 pinch salt

- 1 pinch ground black pepper

- 1 teaspoon distilled white vinegar

- Ground black pepper

DIRECTIONS

1. Preheat oven to 425F or 220C.

2. In a baking dish, place the asparagus and drizzle with the extra-virgin olive oil.

3. In a skillet, heat the olive oil over medium-low heat; add the prosciutto and cook for about 3-4 minutes, stirring until golden and rendered. Sprinkle over the asparagus in the baking dish and season with black pepper; toss to coat.

4. Roast for 10 minutes, stir, return to the oven and continue roasting for 5 minutes or until the asparagus is tender but firm to the bite.

5. Fill a large saucepan with about 2-3 inches of water; bring to a boil over high heat. When boiling, reduce the heat to low; pour in the vinegar and a pinch of salt. Crack an egg into a small bowl, then gently slip the egg into the water. Repeat with the remaining eggs. Poach the eggs for about 4-6 minutes or until the whites are firm and the yolks are thick, but not hard. With a slotted spoon, remove the eggs, dab the spoon on a clean kitchen towel to remove excess water from the eggs, and transfer to a warm plate.

6. Drizzle the asparagus with the lemon juice and transfer divide between o plates. Top each asparagus bed with the o poached eggs, sprinkle with a pinch of lemon zest, and season with black pepper; serve.

NUTRITION Calories 163, Fat 12,3g, Chol 171mg, Sodium 273mg, Carb 4.4g, Fiber 1.9g, Protein 10.4g

Cream Olive Muffins

Servings: 6

Preparation time: 20 minutes

INGREDIENTS

- ½ cup quinoa, cooked

- 2 oz Feta cheese, crumbled

- 2 eggs, beaten

- 3 kalamata olives, chopped

- ¾ cup heavy cream

- 1 tomato, chopped

- 1 teaspoon butter, softened

- 1 tablespoon wheat flour, whole grain

- ½ teaspoon salt

DIRECTIONS

1. In the mixing bowl, whisk eggs and add Feta cheese.

2. Then add chopped tomato and heavy cream.

3. Then add wheat flour, salt, and quinoa.

4. Then add kalamata olives and mix up the ingredients with the help of the spoon.

5. Brush the muffin molds with the butter from inside.

6. Transfer quinoa mixture in the muffin molds and flatten it with the help of the spatula or spoon if needed.

7. Cook the muffins in the preheated to 355F oven for 20 minutes.

NUTRITION Calories 165, Fat 10.8g, Fiber 1.2g, Carbs 11.5g, Protein 5.8g

Veggie Quiche

Servings: 8

Preparation time: 55 minutes

INGREDIENTS

½ cup sun-dried tomatoes, chopped

1 prepared pie crust

2 tablespoons avocado oil

1 yellow onion, chopped

2 garlic cloves, minced

2 cups spinach, chopped

1 red bell pepper, chopped

¼ cup kalamata olives, pitted and sliced

1 teaspoon parsley flakes

1 teaspoon oregano, dried

1/3 cup feta cheese, crumbled

4 eggs, whisked

1 and ½ cups almond milk

1 cup cheddar cheese, shredded

Salt and black pepper to the taste

DIRECTIONS

1. Heat up a pan with the oil over medium-high heat, add the garlic and onion and sauté for 3 minutes.

2. Add the bell pepper and sauté for 3 minutes more.

3. Add the olives, parsley, spinach, oregano, salt, pepper, and cook everything for some minutes.

4. Add tomatoes and the cheese, toss and take off the heat.

5. Arrange the pie crust on a pie plate, pour the spinach and tomatoes mix inside and spread.

6. In a bowl, mix the eggs with salt, pepper, milk, and half of the cheese, whisk and pour over the mixture in the pie crust.

7. Sprinkle the remaining cheese on top and bake at 375 degrees F for 40 minutes.

8. Cool the quiche down, slice, and serve for breakfast.

NUTRITION Calories 211, Fat 14 4g, Fiber 1.4g, Carbs 12.5g, Protein 8.6g

Tuna and Cheese Bake

Servings: 4

Preparation time: 15 minutes

INGREDIENTS

10 ounces canned tuna, drained and flaked

4 eggs, whisked

½ cup feta cheese, shredded

1 tablespoon chives, chopped

1 tablespoon parsley, chopped

Salt and black pepper to the taste

3 teaspoons olive oil

DIRECTIONS

Grease a baking dish with the oil, add the tuna and the rest of the ingredients except the cheese, toss and bake at 370 degrees F for 15 minutes.

Sprinkle the cheese on top, leave the mix aside for 5 minutes, slice, and serve for breakfast.

NUTRITION Calories 283, Fat 14.2g, Fiber 5.6g, Carbs 12.1g, Protein 6.4g

Tomato and Cucumber Salad

Servings: 4

Preparation time: 5 minutes

INGREDIENTS

- 3 tomatoes, chopped

- 2 cucumbers, chopped

- 1 red onion, sliced

- 2 red bell peppers, chopped

- ¼ cup fresh cilantro, chopped

- 1 tablespoon capers

- 1 oz whole-grain bread, chopped

- 1 tablespoon canola oil

- ½ teaspoon minced garlic

- 1 tablespoon Dijon mustard

- 1 teaspoon olive oil

- 1 teaspoon lime juice

DIRECTIONS

Pour canola oil into the skillet and bring it to a boil.

Add chopped bread and roast it until crunchy (3-5 minutes).

Meanwhile, in the salad bowl, combine together sliced red onion, cucumbers, tomatoes, bell peppers, cilantro, capers, and mix up gently.

Make the dressing: mix up together lime juice, olive oil, Dijon mustard, and minced garlic.

Pour the dressing over the salad and stir it directly before serving.

NUTRITION Calories 136, Fat 5.7g, Fiber 4.1g, Carbs 20.2g, Protein 4.1g

Egg and Ham Breakfast Cup

Servings: 12

Preparation time: 12 minutes

INGREDIENTS

- 2 green onion bunch, chopped

- 12 eggs

- 6 thick pieces nitrate free ham

DIRECTIONS

1. Grease a muffin tin and preheat the oven to 400F.

2. Add 2 hams per muffin compartment, press down to form a cup, and add egg in the middle. Repeat the process to the remaining muffin compartments.

3. Pop in the oven and bake until eggs are cooked to desired doneness, around 10 to 12 minutes.

4. To serve, garnish with chopped green onions.

NUTRITION Calories 92, Protein 7.3g, Carbs 0.8g, Fat 6.4g

Eggs Benedict and Artichoke Hearts

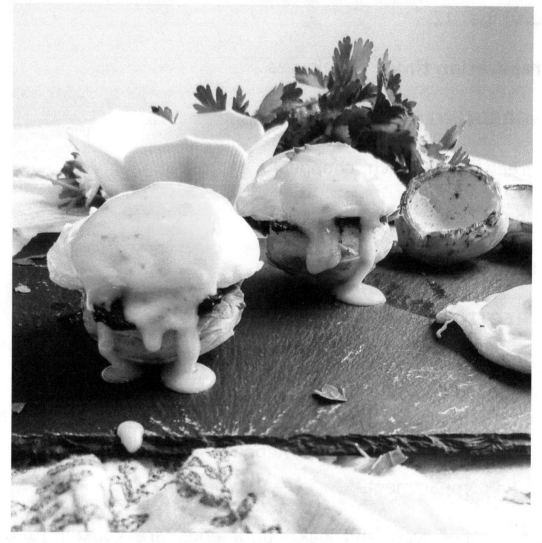

Servings: 2

Preparation time: 30 minutes

INGREDIENTS

Salt and pepper to taste

¾ cup balsamic vinegar

4 artichoke hearts

¼ cup bacon, cooked

1 egg white

8 eggs

1 tablespoon lemon juice

¾ cup melted ghee or butter

DIRECTIONS

Line a baking sheet with parchment paper or foil.

Preheat the oven to 375F.

Deconstruct the artichokes and remove the hearts. Place the hearts in balsamic vinegar for 20 minutes. Set aside.

Prepare the hollandaise sauce by using four eggs and separate the yolk from the white. Reserve the egg white for the artichoke hearts. Add the yolks and lemon juice and cook in a double boiler while stirring constantly to create a silky texture of the sauce. Add the oil and season with salt and pepper. Set aside.

Remove the artichoke hearts from the balsamic vinegar marinade and place them on the cookie sheet. Brush the artichokes with the egg white and cook in the oven for 20 minutes.

6Poach the remaining four eggs. Turn up the heat and let the water boil. Crack the eggs one at a time and cook for a minute before removing the egg.

Assemble by layering the artichokes, bacon, and poached eggs.

Pour over the hollandaise sauce.

Serve with toasted bread.

NUTRITION Calories: 640; Protein: 28 3g: Carbs: 36.0g; Fat: 42.5g

Creamy Frittata

Servings: 4

Preparation time: 15 minutes

INGREDIENTS

- 5 eggs, beaten

- 1 poblano chile, chopped, raw

- 1 oz scallions, chopped

- 1/3 cup heavy cream

- ½ teaspoon butter

- ½ teaspoon salt

- ½ teaspoon chili flakes

- 1 tablespoon fresh cilantro, chopped

DIRECTIONS

Mix up together eggs with heavy cream and whisk until homogenous.

Add chopped poblano chile, scallions, salt, chili flakes, and fresh cilantro.

Toss butter in the skillet and melt it.

Add egg mixture and flatten it in the skillet if needed.

Close the lid and cook the frittata for 15 minutes over medium-low heat.

When the frittata is cooked, it will be solid.

NUTRITION Calories 131, Fat 10.4g, Fiber 0.2g, Carbs 1.3g, Protein 8.2g

Dill, Havarti & Asparagus Frittata

Servings: 4

Preparation time: 20 minutes

INGREDIENTS

- 1 tsp dried dill weed or 2 tsp minced fresh dill

- 4 oz Havarti cheese cut into small cubes

- 6 eggs, beaten welt

- Pepper and salt to taste

- 1 stalk green onions sliced for garnish

- 3 tsp. olive oil

- 2/3 cup diced cherry tomatoes

- 6-8 oz fresh asparagus, ends trimmed and cut into 1 ½-inch length

DIRECTIONS

1. Over medium-high fire, place a large cast-iron pan and add oil. Once the oil is hot, stir-fry asparagus for 4 minutes.

2. Add dill weed and tomatoes. Cook for two minutes.

3. Meanwhile, season eggs with pepper and salt. Beat well.

4. Pour eggs over the tomatoes.

5. Evenly spread cheese on top.

6. Preheat broiler.

7. Lower the fire to low, cover the pan, and let it cook for 10 minutes until the cheese on top has melted.

8. Turn off the fire and transfer the pan to the oven and broil for 2 minutes or until the tops are browned.

9. Remove from the oven, sprinkle sliced green onions, serve, and enjoy.

   NUTRITIONAL Calories per service: 244, Protein: 16g; Carbs: 3.7g: Fat: 18.3g

Egg and Pepper Bake

Servings: 4

Preparation time: 28 minutes

INGREDIENTS

- 2 eggs, beaten

- 1 red bell pepper, chopped

- 1 chili pepper, chopped

- ½ red onion, diced

- 1 teaspoon canola oil

- ½ teaspoon salt

- 1 teaspoon paprika

- 1 tablespoon fresh cilantro, chopped

- 1 garlic clove, diced

- 1 teaspoon butter, softened

- ¼ teaspoon chili flakes

DIRECTIONS

Brush the casserole mold with canola oil and pour beaten eggs inside.

Then toss the butter in the skillet and melt it over medium heat.

Add chili pepper and red bell pepper.

Then, add red onion and cook the vegetables for 7-8 minutes over medium heat. Stir them from time to time.

Transfer the vegetables to the casserole mold.

Add salt, paprika, cilantro, diced garlic, and chili flakes. Stir gently with the help of a spatula to get a homogenous mixture.

Bake the casserole for no minutes at 355F in the oven.

Then chill the meal well and cut into servings. Transfer the casserole to the serving plates with the help of the spatula.

NUTRITION Calories 68, Fat 4.5g, Fiber 1g, Carbs 4.4g, Protein 3.4g

Mediterranean Chicken Salad Pitas

Servings: 6

Preparation time: 15 minutes

INGREDIENTS

- 6 pieces (6-inch) whole-wheat pitas, cut into halves

- 6 slices (1/8-inch-thick) tomato, cut into halves

- 1 can (15-ounce) chickpeas (garbanzo beans), no-salt-added, rinsed, drained

- 3 cups chicken, cooked, chopped

- 2 tablespoons lemon juice

- 12 Bibb lettuce leaves

- ¼ teaspoon red pepper, crushed

- ¼ cup fresh cilantro, chopped

- ½ teaspoon ground cumin

- ½ cup red onion, diced

- ½ cup (about 20 small) green olives, chopped, pitted

- 1 cup Greek yogurt, plain, whole-milk

- 1 cup (about 1 large) red bell pepper, chopped

DIRECTIONS

1. In a small bowl, combine the yogurt, lemon juice, cumin, and red pepper; set aside.

2. In a large mixing bowl, combine the chicken, red bell pepper, olives, red onion, cilantro, and chickpeas. Add the yogurt mixture into the chicken mixture; gently toss to coat.

3. Line each pita half with 1 lettuce leaf and then with 1 tomato slice. Fill each pita half with ½ cup of the chicken mixture.

NUTRITION Calories 404, Fat 10.2g, Chol 66mg, Sodium 575mg, Carb 46.4g, Fiber 6g, Protein 33.6g

Raspberries and Yogurt Smoothie

Servings: 2

Preparation time: 0 minutes

INGREDIENTS

- 2 cups raspberries

- ½ cup Greek yogurt

- ½ cup almond milk

- ½ teaspoon vanilla extract

DIRECTIONS

In your blender, combine the raspberries with the milk, vanilla, and the yogurt, pulse well, divide into 2 glasses and serve for breakfast.

NUTRITION Calories 245, Fat 9.5g, Fiber 2.3g, Carbs 5.6g, Protein 1.6g

Breakfast Spanakopita

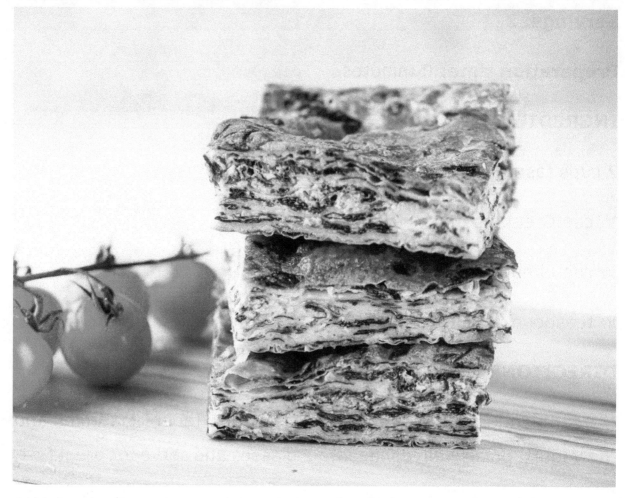

Servings: 6

Preparation time: 1 Hour

INGREDIENTS

- 2 cups spinach

- 1 white onion, diced

- ½ cup fresh parsley

- 1 teaspoon minced garlic

- 3 oz Feta cheese, crumbled

- 1 teaspoon ground paprika

- 2 eggs, beaten

- 1/3 cup butter, melted

- 2 oz Phyllo dough

DIRECTIONS

Separate Phyllo dough into 2 parts.

Brush the casserole mold with butter well and place 1 part of Phyllo dough inside.

Brush its surface with butter too.

Put the spinach and fresh parsley in the blender. Blend it until smooth and transfer in the mixing bowl.

Add minced garlic, Feta cheese, ground paprika, eggs, and diced onion. Mix up well.

Place the spinach mixture in the casserole mold and flatten it well.

Cover the spinach mixture with the remaining Phyllo dough and pour the remaining butter over it.

Bake spanakopita for 1 hour at 350F.

Cut it into servings.

NUTRITION Calories 190, Fat 15.4g, Fiber 1.1g, Carbs 8.4g, Protein 5.4g

Farro Salad

Servings: 2

Preparation time: 4 minutes

INGREDIENTS

- 1 tablespoon olive oil

- A pinch of salt and black pepper

- 1 bunch baby spinach, chopped

- 1 avocado, pitted, peeled, and chopped

- 1 garlic clove, minced

- 2 cups farro, already cooked

- ½ cup cherry tomatoes, cubed

DIRECTIONS

1. Heat up a pan with the oil over medium heat, add the spinach, and the rest of the ingredients, toss, cook for 4 minutes, divide into bowls and serve.

   NUTRITION Calories 157, Fat 13.7g, Fiber 5.5g, Carbs 8.6g, Protein 3.6g

Chili Avocado Scramble

Servings: 4

Preparation time: 15 minutes

INGREDIENTS

4 eggs, beaten

1 white onion, diced

1 tablespoon avocado oil

1 avocado, finely chopped

½ teaspoon chili flakes

1 oz Cheddar cheese, shredded

½ teaspoon salt

1 tablespoon fresh parsley

DIRECTIONS

1. Pour avocado oil into the skillet and bring it to a boil.

2. Then add diced onion and roast it until it is light brown.

3. Meanwhile, mix up together chili flakes, beaten eggs, and salt.

4. Pour the egg mixture over the cooked onion and cook the mixture for 1 minute over medium heat.

5. Then, scramble the eggs well with the help of the fork or spatula. Cook the eggs until they are solid but soft.

6. Then, add chopped avocado and shredded cheese.

7. Stir well and transfer in the serving plates.

8. Sprinkle the meal with fresh parsley.

   NUTRITION Calories 236, Fat 20.1g, Fiber 4g, Carbs 7.4g, Protein 8.6g

Tapioca Pudding

Servings: 3

Preparation time: 15 minutes

INGREDIENTS

* ¼ cup pearl tapioca

* ¼ cup maple syrup

* 2 cups almond milk

* ½ cup coconut flesh, shredded

* 1 and ½ teaspoon lemon juice

DIRECTIONS

In a pan, combine the milk with the tapioca and the rest of the ingredients, bring to a simmer over medium heat and cook for 15 minutes.

Divide the mix into bowls, cool it down, and serve for breakfast.

NUTRITION Calories 361, Fat 28.5g, Fiber 2.7g, Carbs 28.3g, Protein 2.8g

Ricotta Tartine and Honey Roasted Cherry

Servings: 4

Preparation time: 15 minutes

INGREDIENTS

- 4 slices (1/2 inch thick) artisan bread, whole-grain

- 2 cups fresh cherries, pitted

- 2 teaspoons extra-virgin olive oil

- ¼ cup slivered almonds, toasted

- 1 teaspoon lemon zest

- 1 teaspoon fresh thyme

- 1 tablespoon lemon juice

- 1 tablespoon honey, plus more for serving

- 1 cup ricotta cheese, part-skim

- Pinch of flaky sea salt, such as Maldon

- Pinch of salt

DIRECTIONS

1. Preheat oven to 400F. Line a rimmed baking sheet with parchment paper; set aside.

2. In a mixing bowl, toss the cherries with the honey, oil, lemon juice, and salt. Transfer into a pan. Roast for about 15 minutes, shaking the pan once or twice during roasting until the cherries are very soft and warm.

3. Toast the bread. Top with the cheese, cherries, thyme, lemon zest, almonds, and season with sea salt. If desired, drizzle more honey.

NUTRITION Calories 320, Fat 13g, Carb 39g, Fiber 6g, Sugar 2g, Protein 15g

Mediterranean Breakfast Quiche

Servings: 1/8 Quiche

Preparation time: 1 Hour

INGREDIENTS

- 11/2 cups all-purpose flour

- 1 tsp. dried oregano

- ½ tsp. garlic powder

- 2 tsp. salt

- 5 TB. cold butter

- 3 TB. vegetable shortening

- ¼ cup ice water

- 3 TB. extra-virgin olive oil

- 1 medium yellow onion, chopped

- 1 TB. minced garlic

- 4 stalks asparagus, chopped

- 2 cups spinach, chopped

- 4 large eggs

- ½ cup heavy cream

- 1 cup ricotta cheese

- 1/3 cup grated Parmesan cheese

- 1 tsp. paprika

- ½ tsp. cayenne

- ½ tsp. ground black pepper

- ¼ cup fresh basil, chopped

- ¼ cup fresh parsley, chopped

- 1/3 cup sun-dried tomatoes, chopped

DIRECTIONS

1. In a food processor fitted with a chopping blade, pulse together 11/2 cups all-purpose flour, oregano, garlic powder, and ½ teaspoon salt five times.

2. Add cold butter and vegetable shortening, and pulse for 1 minute or until mixture resembles coarse meal.

3. Continue to pulse while adding ice water, about 1 minute. Test dough if it holds together when you pinch it, it doesn't need any more water.

4. If it doesn't come together, add 3 more tablespoons of cold water.

5. Remove dough from the food processor, put it into a plastic bag, and form into a flat disc. Refrigerate for 3 minutes.

6. Preheat the oven to 400°F. Flour a rolling pin and your counter.

7. Roll out dough to ¼ inch thickness. Fit dough into an 8- or 9-inch tart pan. Using a fork, slightly puncture the bottom of the piecrust. Bake for 15 minutes. Remove from the oven and set aside.

8. In a large skillet over medium heat, add extra-virgin olive oil, yellow onion, garlic, and asparagus, and sauté for 5 minutes.

9. Add spinach and cook for 3 or 4 more minutes. Remove from heat and set aside.

10.   In a large bowl, whisk together eggs, heavy cream, and ricotta cheese.

11.   Add remaining teaspoons of salt, Parmesan cheese, paprika, cayenne, black pepper, basil, parsley, and sun-dried tomatoes, and stir to combine.

12.   Pour filling into the piecrust, and bake for 4 minutes. Remove from the oven, and let rest for no minutes before serving warm.

NUTRITION Calories 346, Fat 19.4g, Protein 14.9g, Chol 34mg, Sodium 767mg, Pot 998mg

Feta and Eggs Mix

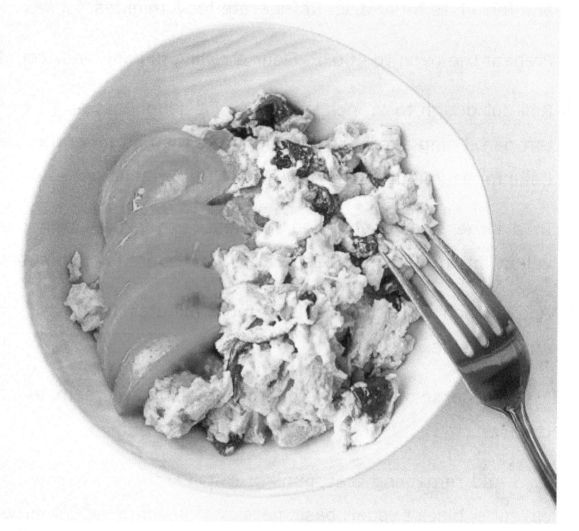

Servings: 4

Preparation time: 5 minutes

INGREDIENTS

- 4 eggs, beaten

- ½ teaspoon ground black pepper

- 2 oz Feta, scrambled

- ½ teaspoon salt

- 1 teaspoon butter

- 1 teaspoon fresh parsley, chopped

DIRECTIONS

1. Melt butter in the skillet and add beaten eggs.

2. Then add parsley, salt, and scrambled eggs. Cook the eggs for 1 minute over high heat.

3. Add ground black pepper and scrambled eggs with the help of the fork.

4. Cook the eggs for 3 minutes over medium-high heat.

   NUTRITION Calories 110, Fat 8.4g, Fiber 0.1g, Carbs 1.1g, Protein 7.6g

Creamy Parsley Soufflé

Servings: 2

Preparation time: **25 minutes**

INGREDIENTS

- 2 fresh red chili peppers, chopped

- Salt to taste

- 4 eggs

- 4 tablespoons light cream

- 2 tablespoons fresh parsley, chopped

DIRECTIONS

1. Preheat the oven to 375 degrees F and grease o soufflé dishes.

2. Combine all the ingredients in a bowl and mix well.

3. Put the mixture into prepared soufflé dishes and transfer it to the oven.

4. Cook for about 6 minutes and dish out to serve immediately.

5. For meal preparation, you can refrigerate this creamy parsley soufflé in the ramekins covered in a foil for about 2-3 days.

NUTRITION Calories: 108 Fat: 9g Carbohydrates: 1.1g Protein: 6g

Betty Oats

Servings: 2

Preparation time: 0 minutes

INGREDIENTS

½ cup rolled oats

1 cup almond milk

¼ cup chia seeds

A pinch of cinnamon powder

2 teaspoons honey

1 cup berries, pureed

1 tablespoon yogurt

DIRECTIONS

In a bowl, combine the oats with the milk and the rest of the ingredients except the yogurt, toss, divide into bowls, top with the yogurt and serve cold for breakfast.

NUTRITION Calories 420, Fat 30.3g, Fiber 7.2g, Carbs 35.3g, Protein 6.4g

Zucchini Oats

Servings: 4

Preparation time: 20 minutes

INGREDIENTS

- 2 cups rolled oats

- 2 cups of water

- ½ teaspoon salt

- 1 tablespoon butter

- 1 zucchini, grated

- ¼ teaspoon ground ginger

DIRECTIONS

1. Pour water into the saucepan.

2. Add rolled oats, butter, and salt.

3. Stir gently and start to cook the oats for 4 minutes over high heat.

4. When the mixture starts to boil, add ground ginger and grated zucchini. Stir well.

5. Cook the oats for some minutes over medium-low heat.

NUTRITION Calories 189, Fat 5.7g, Fiber 4.7g, Carbs 29.4g, Protein 6g

Spinach Artichoke Egg Casserole

Servings: 2

Preparation time: 45 minutes

INGREDIENTS

1/8 cup milk

2.5-ounce frozen chopped spinach, thawed and drained well

1/8 cup parmesan cheese

1/8 cup onions, shaved

¼ teaspoon salt

¼ teaspoon crushed red pepper

4 large eggs

3 5-ounce artichoke hearts, drained

¼ cup white cheddar, shredded

1/8 cup ricotta cheese

½ garlic clove, minced

¼ teaspoon dried thyme

DIRECTIONS

1. Preheat the oven to 350 degrees F and grease a baking dish with non-stick cooking spray.

2. Whisk eggs and milk together and add artichoke hearts and spinach.

3. Mix well and stir in the rest of the ingredients, withholding the ricotta cheese.

4. Pour the mixture into the baking dish and top evenly with ricotta cheese.

5. Transfer in the oven and bake for about 3 minutes.

6. Dish out and serve warm.

NUTRITION Calories:228 Carbs: 10.1g Fat: 13.3g Protein: 19.1g Sodium: 571mg Sugar: 2.5g

Avocado Chickpea Pizza

Servings: 2

Preparation time: 20 minutes

INGREDIENTS

1 and ¼ cups chickpea flour

A pinch of salt and black pepper

1 and ¼ cups water

2 tablespoons olive oil

1 teaspoon onion powder

1 teaspoon garlic, minced

1 tomato, sliced

1 avocado, peeled, pitted, and sliced

2 ounces gouda, sliced

¼ cup tomato sauce

2 tablespoons green onions, chopped

DIRECTIONS

1. In a bowl, mix the chickpea flour with salt, pepper, water, oil, onion powder, and garlic, stir well until you obtain a dough, knead a bit, put in a bowl, cover, and leave aside for no minutes.

2. Transfer the dough to a working surface, shape a bit circle, transfer it to a baking sheet lined with parchment paper and bake at 425 degrees F for 10 minutes.

3. Spread the tomato sauce over the pizza, also spread the rest of the ingredients, and bake at 400 degrees F for 10 minutes more.

4. Cut and serve for breakfast.

NUTRITION Calories 416, Fat 24.5g, Fiber 9.6g, Carbs 36.6g, Protein 15.4g

Avocado Milk Shake

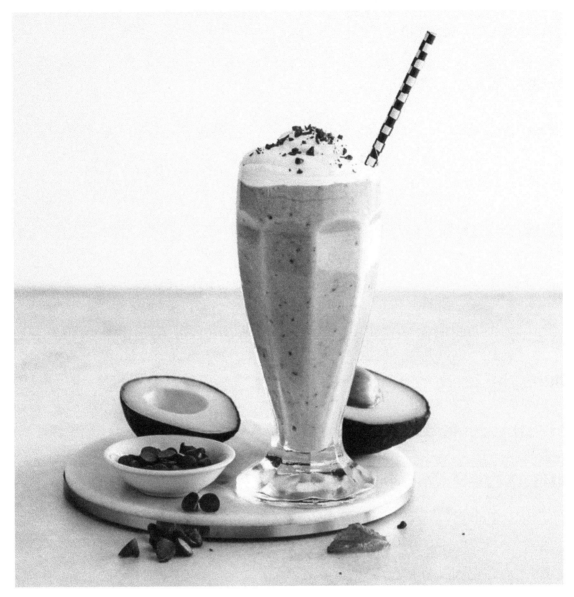

Servings: 3

Preparation time: 10 minutes

INGREDIENTS

1 avocado, peeled, pitted

2 tablespoons of liquid honey

½ teaspoon vanilla extract

½ cup heavy cream

1 cup milk

1/ 3 cup ice cubes

DIRECTIONS

1. Chop the avocado and put it in the food processor.

2. Add liquid honey, vanilla extract, heavy cream, milk, and ice cubes.

3. Blend the mixture until it is smooth.

4. Pour the cooked milkshake into the serving glasses.

NUTRITION Calories 291, Fat 22.1g, Fiber 4.5g, Carbs 22g, Protein 4.4g

Pizza with Sprouts

Servings: 6

Preparation time: 35 minutes

INGREDIENTS

- ½ cup wheat flour, whole grain

- 2 tablespoons butter, softened

- ¼ teaspoon baking powder

- ¾ teaspoon salt

- 5 oz chicken fillet, boiled

- 2 oz Cheddar cheese, shredded

- 1 teaspoon tomato sauce

- 1 oz bean sprouts

DIRECTIONS

Make the pizza crust: mix up together wheat flour, butter, baking powder, and salt. Knead the soft and non-sticky dough. Add more wheat flour if needed.

Leave the dough for 10 minutes to chill.

Then place the dough on the baking paper. Cover it with the second baking paper sheet.

Roll up the dough with the help of the rolling pin to get the round pizza crust.

After this, remove the upper baking paper sheet.

Transfer the pizza crust to the tray.

Spread the crust with tomato sauce.

Then shred the chicken fillet and arrange it over the pizza crust.

Add shredded Cheddar cheese.

Bake pizza for 20 minutes at 355F.

Then top the cooked pizza with bean sprouts and slice it into servings.

NUTRITION Calories 157, Fat 8.8g, Fiber 0.3g, Carbs 8.4g, Protein 10.5g

Feta and Quinoa Egg Muffins

Servings: 12

Preparation time: 30 minutes

INGREDIENTS

- 8 eggs

- 2 teaspoons olive oil

- 2 cups baby spinach, finely chopped

- ¼ teaspoon salt

- ½ cup onion, finely chopped

- ½ cup kalamata olives, chopped, pitted

- 1 tablespoon fresh oregano, chopped

- 1 cup quinoa*, cooked

- 1 cup grape or cherry tomatoes, sliced or chopped

- 1 cup feta cheese, crumbled

DIRECTIONS

Preheat oven to 350F.

Grease a 12 muffin with oil or place in silicone muffin holders on a baking sheet.

Heat a skillet over medium heat. Add the olive oil. Add onions; sauté for about 2 minutes. Add the tomatoes, sauté for 1 minute more. Add the spinach; sauté for about 1 minute or until wilted. Turn the heat off.

Stir in the olives and the oregano; set aside.

Put the eggs in a bowl and whisk. Add the feta, quinoa, vegetable mixture, and salt; stir until well mixed. Pour the mixture into the prepared muffin tins or silicone cups, dividing equally; bake for about 3 minutes or until the eggs are set and light golden brown. Cool for 5 minutes and then serve. You can eat these warm, chilled, or cold. To reheat leftovers, just microwave.

NUTRITION Calories 120, Fat 3g, Carb 6g, Fiber 1g, Sugar 2g, Protein 7g

Cauliflower Skillet

Servings: 5

Preparation time: 25 minutes

INGREDIENTS

1 cup cauliflower, chopped

1 tablespoon olive oil

½ red onion, diced

1 tablespoon Plain yogurt

½ teaspoon ground black pepper

1 teaspoon dried cilantro

1 teaspoon dried oregano

1 bell pepper, chopped

1/ 3 cup milk

½ teaspoon Za'atar

1 tablespoon lemon juice

1 russet potato, chopped

DIRECTIONS

1. Pour olive oil into the skillet and preheat it.

2. Add chopped russet potato and roast it for 5 minutes.

3. Then, add cauliflower, ground black pepper, cilantro, oregano, and bell pepper.

4. Roast the mixture for 10 minutes over medium heat. Then add milk, Za'atar, and Plain Yogurt. Stir it well.

5. Saute the mixture for 10 minutes.

6. Top the cooked meal with diced red onion and sprinkle with lemon juice.

7. It is recommended to serve the breakfast hot.

NUTRITION Calories 112, Fat 3.4g, Fiber 2.6g, Carbs 18.1g, Protein 3.1g

Cheese Pies

Servings: 6

Preparation time: 20 minutes

INGREDIENTS

- 7 OZ yufka dough/phyllo dough

- 1 cup Cheddar cheese, shredded

- 1 cup fresh cilantro, chopped

- 2 eggs, beaten

- 1 teaspoon paprika

- ¼ teaspoon chili flakes

- ½ teaspoon salt

- 2 tablespoons sour cream

- 1 teaspoon olive oil

DIRECTION

In the mixing bowl, combine together sour cream, salt, chili flakes, paprika, and beaten eggs.

Brush the springform pan with olive oil.

Place ¼ part of all yufka dough in the pan and sprinkle it with ¼ part of the egg mixture.

Add a ¼ cup of cheese and ¼ cup of cilantro.

Cover the mixture with 1/3 part of the remaining yufka dough and repeat all the steps again. You should get 4 layers.

Cut the yufka mixture into 6 pies and bake at 360F for 20 minutes.

The cooked pies should have a golden brown color.

NUTRITION Calories 213, Fat 11.4g, Fiber 0.8g, Carbs 18.2g, Protein 9.1g

Spinach Pie

Servings: 6

Preparation time: 1 Hour

INGREDIENTS

- 2 cups spinach

- 1 white onion, diced

- ½ cup fresh parsley

- 1 teaspoon minced garlic

- 3 oz Feta cheese, crumbled

- 1 teaspoon ground paprika o eggs, beaten

- 1/3 cup butter, melted

- 2 oz Phyllo dough

DIRECTIONS

1. Separate Phyllo dough into 2 parts.

2. Brush the casserole mold with butter well and place 1 part of Phyllo dough inside.

3. Brush its surface with butter too.

4. Put the spinach and fresh parsley in the blender. Blend it until smooth and transfer in the mixing bowl.

5. Add minced garlic, Feta cheese, ground paprika, eggs, and diced onion. Mix up well.

6. Place the spinach mixture in the casserole mold and flatten it well.

7. Cover the spinach mixture with the remaining Phyllo dough and pour the remaining butter over it.

8. Bake spanakopita for 1 hour at 350F.

9. Cut it into servings.

NUTRITION Calories 190, Fat 15.4g, Fiber 1.1g, Carbs 8.4g, Protein 5.4g

Bacon, Spinach and Tomato Sandwich

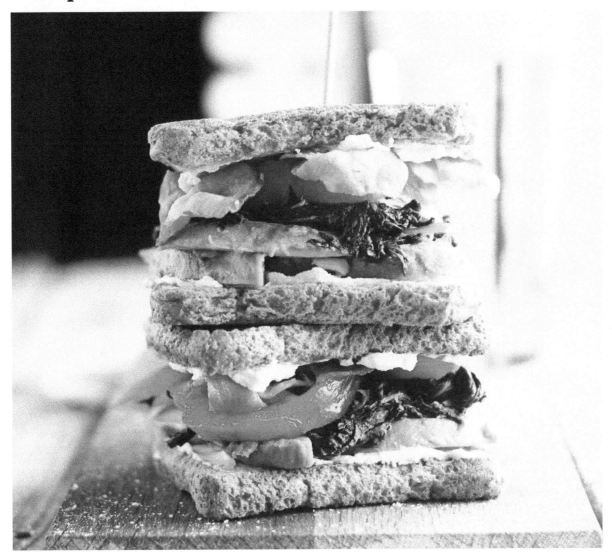

Servings: 1

Preparation time: 0 minutes

INGREDIENTS

- 2 whole-wheat bread slices, toasted

- 1 tablespoon Dijon mustard

- 3 bacon slices

- Salt and black pepper to the taste

- 2 tomato slices

- ¼ cup baby spinach

DIRECTIONS

Spread the mustard on each bread slice, divide the bacon and the rest of the ingredients on one slice, top with the other one, cut in half, and serve for breakfast.

NUTRITION Calories 246, Fat 11.2g, Fiber 4.5g, Carbs 17.5g, Protein 8.3g

Open-Face Egg and Bacon Sandwich

Servings: 1

Preparation time: 20 minutes

INGREDIENTS

- ¼ oz reduced-fat cheddar, shredded

- ½ small jalapeno, thinly sliced

- ½ whole-grain English muffin, split

- 1 large organic egg

- 1 thick slice of tomato

- 1-piece turkey bacon

- 2 thin slices red onion

- 4-5 sprigs fresh cilantro

- Cooking spray

- Pepper to taste

DIRECTIONS

On medium fire, place a skillet, cook bacon until crisp-tender, and set aside.

In the same skillet, drain oils, and place ½ of English muffin and heat for at least a minute per side. Transfer muffin to a serving plate.

Coat the same skillet with cooking spray and fry an egg to the desired doneness. Once cooked, place the egg on top of the muffin.

Add cilantro, tomato, onion, jalapeno, and bacon on top of the egg. Serve and enjoy

NUTRITION Calories 245, Carbs 24.7g, Protein 11.8g, Fat 11g

Watermelon Pizza

Servings: 2

Preparation time: 10 minutes

INGREDIENTS

- 9 oz watermelon slice

- 1 tablespoon Pomegranate sauce

- 2 oz Feta cheese, crumbled

- 1 tablespoon fresh cilantro, chopped

DIRECTIONS

Place the watermelon slice on the plate and sprinkle it with crumbled Feta cheese.

Add fresh cilantro.

Then, sprinkle the pizza with Pomegranate juice generously.

Cut the pizza into servings.

NUTRITION Calories 143, Fat 6.2g, Fiber 0.6g, Carbs 18 .4g, Protein 5.1g

Artichokes and Cheese Omelet

Servings: 1

Preparation time: 8 minutes

INGREDIENTS

1 teaspoon avocado oil

1 tablespoon almond milk

2 eggs, whisked

A pinch of salt and black pepper

2 tablespoons tomato, cubed

2 tablespoons kalamata olives, pitted and sliced

1 artichoke heart, chopped

1 tablespoon tomato sauce

1 tablespoon feta cheese, crumbled

DIRECTIONS

In a bowl, combine the eggs with the milk, salt, pepper, and the rest of the ingredients except the avocado oil and whisk well.

Heat up a pan with the avocado oil over medium-high heat, add the omelet mix, spread into the pan, cook for 4 minutes, flip, cook for 4 minutes more, transfer to a plate, and serve.

NUTRITION Calories 303, Fat 17.7g, Fiber 9.9g, Carbs 21.9g, Protein 18.2g

Parmesan Omelet

Servings: 2

Preparation time: 15 minutes

INGREDIENTS

- 1 tablespoon cream cheese

- 2 eggs, beaten

- ¼ teaspoon paprika

- ½ teaspoon dried oregano

- ¼ teaspoon dried dill

- 1 oz Parmesan, grated

- 1 teaspoon coconut oil

DIRECTIONS

1. Mix up together cream cheese with eggs, dried oregano, and dill.

2. Put the coconut oil in the pan and heat it until it covers the entire pan.

3. Then pour the egg mixture into the skillet and flatten it.

4. Add grated Parmesan and close the lid.

5. Cook omelet for 10 minutes over low heat.

6. Then transfer the cooked omelet to the serving plate and sprinkle with paprika.

   NUTRITION: Calories 148, Fat 11.5g, Fiber 0.3g, Carbs 1.4g, Protein 10.6g

Creamy Oatmeal with Figs

Servings: 5

Preparation time: 30 minutes

INGREDIENTS

- 2 cups oatmeal

- 1 ½ cup milk

- 1 tablespoon butter

- 3 figs, chopped

- 1 tablespoon honey

DIRECTIONS

Pour milk into the saucepan.

Add oatmeal and close the lid.

Cook the oatmeal for 15 minutes over medium-low heat.

Then add chopped figs and honey.

Add butter and mix up the oatmeal well.

Cook it for 5 minutes more.

Close the lid and let the cooked breakfast rest for 10 minutes before serving.

NUTRITION Calories 222, Fat 6g, Fiber 4.4g, Carbs 36.5g, Protein 7.1g

Conclusion

We've come to the end of this beautiful journey, there may have been some difficulties, but I hope you've enjoyed these tasty and healthy lunches to the fullest.

What have your relatives told you?

Have you been practising your cooking?

If they haven't come out perfect yet, don't get discouraged and keep practicing all the time.

I'm sure you will become very good at it.

I hug you and thank you ... see you on the next culinary journey.

CPSIA information can be obtained
at www.ICGtesting.com
Printed in the USA
BVHW061014130421
604814BV00008B/1362